PARKINSON'S DISEASE

Published by Smart Apple Media
1980 Lookout Drive
North Mankato, Minnesota 56003

Copyright © 2001 Smart Apple Media.
International copyrights reserved in all countries.
No part of this book may be reproduced in any form without
written permission from the publisher.
Printed in the United States of America.

Photos: pages 7, 15—LifeART, Lippincott Williams & Wilkins;
page 9—Indexstock: Michael Howell; page 10—Allsport UK/ALL-
SPORT; page 11—Matthew Mendelsohn/CORBIS; pages 14, 17—
Indexstock: BSIP Agency, page 18—Indexstock: Jacob Halaska;
page 22—Indexstock: Lonnie Duka; page 24—Indexstock: Stew-
art Cohen; page 27—Dr. Robert A. Bloodgood, University of
Virginia School of Medicine; page 29—AFP/CORBIS

Design and Production: EvansDay Design

Library of Congress Cataloging-in-Publication Data

Vander Hook, Sue, 1949–
Parkinson's disease / by Sue Vander Hook
p. cm. – (Understanding illness)
Includes index.
Summary: Describes Parkinson's disease, including the history of
its discovery and profiles of those who survive and cope with it.
ISBN 1-58340-055-9
1. Parkinson's disease—Juvenile literature. [1. Parkinson's dis-
ease. 2. Diseases.] I. Title. II. Series: Understanding illness
(Mankato, Minn.)

RC382.V34   2000
616.8'33—dc21   99-29939

First edition

9 8 7 6 5 4 3 2 1

UNDERSTANDING ILLNESS

PARKINSON'S DISEASE

Sue Vander Hook

The HUMAN BRAIN

THAN THE MOST ADVANCED COMPUTER.

Connected to a network of nerves, the brain is responsible for everything the body does, including walking, talking, eating, and reacting to pain. When even a tiny portion of the brain is not functioning correctly, messages sent to the body may become scrambled. Movements may become slow, one side of the body may experience tremors, limbs and muscles may stiffen, and walking may become difficult. This communication problem between the brain and the body is a condition known as Parkinson's disease.

IS MORE COMPLEX

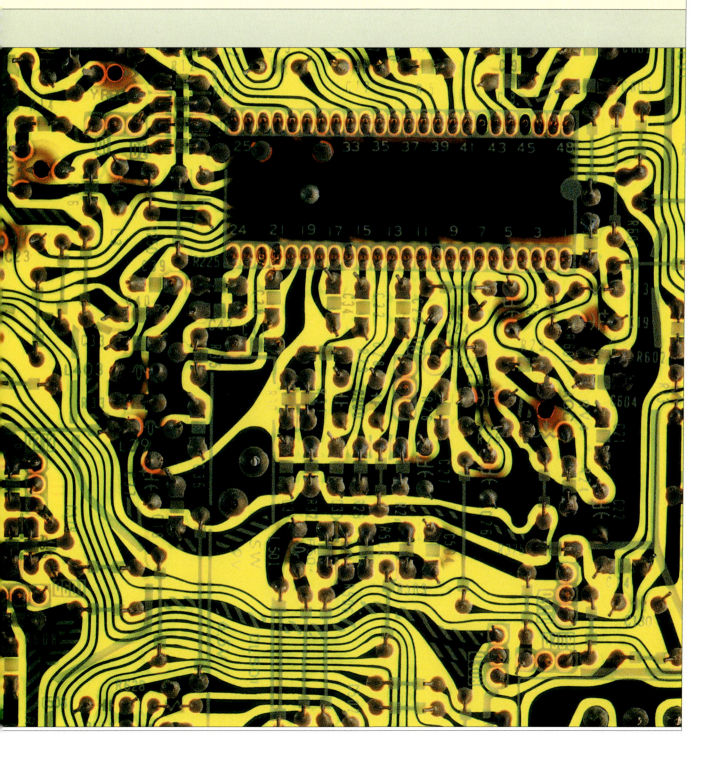

WHAT'S IN A BRAIN?

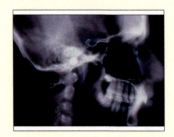

Parkinson's is described as a **chronic** disease. Once people have Parkinson's, they have it for the rest of their lives since there is no known cure. It is important to note, however, that Parkinson's is neither contagious nor fatal. Even though it is defined as a **neurological** condition, the disease does not actually damage the

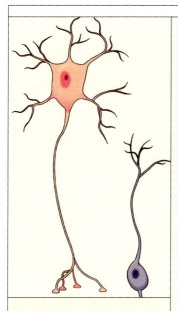

An illustration of a neuron. Billions of these brain cells help us to think and move.

chronic: continuing over a long time

neurological: relating to the nervous system

The middle section of the human brain acts as a control center, telling muscles what to do when we want to move.

nerves, but damages cells in the brain called neurons. Billions of neurons control everything a person does. One type of neuron controls thoughts, while another kind is in charge of the **senses**. Other neurons regulate a person's breathing, heart rate, and other **involuntary** functions such as digestion.

The control center for voluntary body movements is located in a part of the midbrain called the *basal ganglia*. Special neurons in

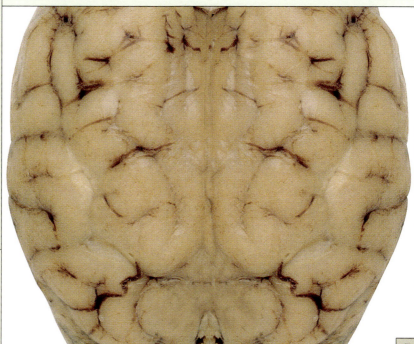

this area are always ready to help the body move quickly and smoothly. When a person wants to raise his arm, messages are sent immediately from the basal ganglia to muscles in the shoulder, elbow, wrist, hand, and any other parts that need to help lift the arm.

The message is first triggered by a chemical **transmitter** called dopamine. In an area of the

senses: the functions of sight, hearing, smell, taste, and touch

involuntary: occurring without choice or control

Our brains transmit the chemical dopamine, which allows us to coordinate the movements of many muscles at once.

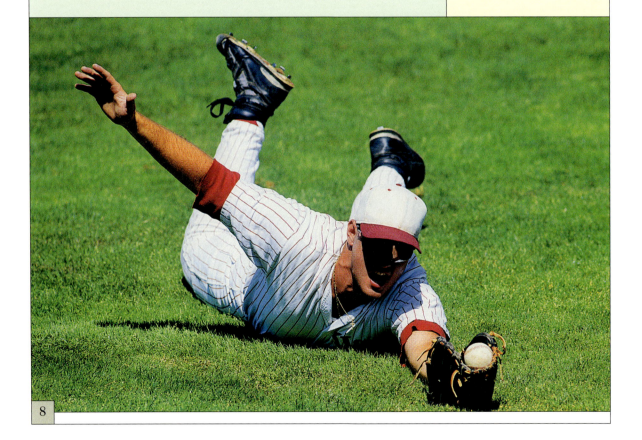

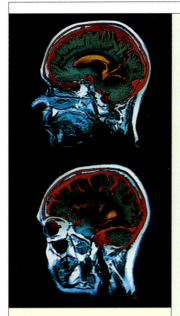

Images called brain scans let doctors look directly at a person's brain and skull structure.

basal ganglia called the *substantia nigra*, special **nigral** cells are constantly making dopamine. When released, dopamine communicates with other parts of the brain also involved in controlling movement. If these nigral cells die, less dopamine is produced in the brain, eventually resulting in Parkinson's disease. As more nigral cells are destroyed, the symptoms of the disease become worse. With less and less dopamine telling the body how to move, a person's movements become slower and less controlled.

transmitter: something that sends signals or messages from one place to another

nigral: relating to an area of the brain called the substantia nigra

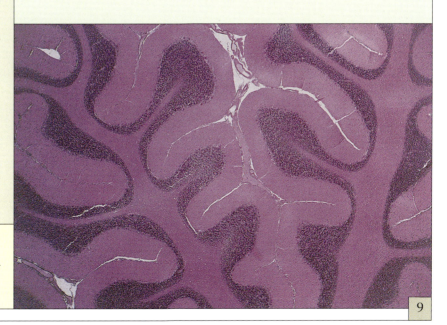

This microscopic image shows the brain cells of a person with Parkinson's disease.

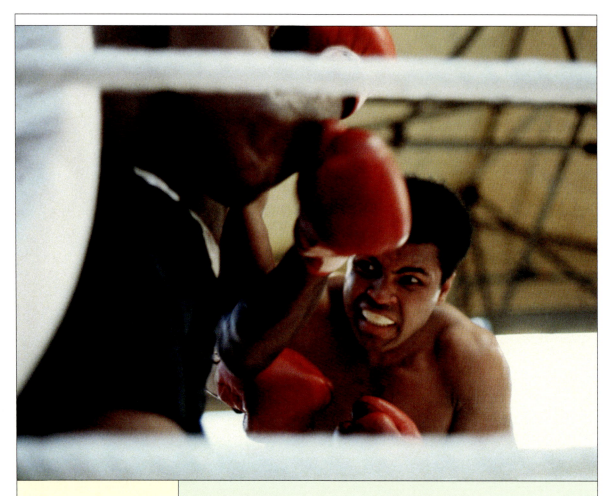

Boxing legend Muhammad Ali has Parkinson's. Some people believe it was caused by taking so many punches to the head.

degeneration: the worsening of a quality or condition

Degeneration of nigral cells is gradual, making Parkinson's a **progressive** disease. Cell death leading to Parkinson's can be caused by several things, including severe injury to the head, infection, poisoning, and other neurological diseases. Some drugs interfere with the brain's ability to use dopamine, causing Parkinson's symptoms. Usually, scientists do not know exactly why nigral cells are lost or destroyed. Although Parkinson's usually strikes people over the age of 60, it is possible for younger people to develop the disease as well. About 10 percent of people with Parkinson's disease are under 40 years old.

progressive: moving onward step by step

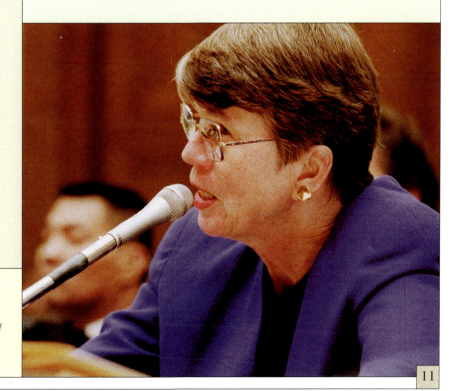

Despite living with Parkinson's, Janet Reno has had a successful career as the Attorney General of the United States.

JOURNEY TO THE CENTER OF THE BRAIN

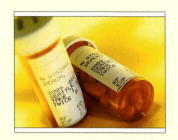

Over time, drugs used to treat Parkinson's may become less and less effective, and other treatments may become necessary. One option may be a surgery called a pallidotomy. To perform this operation, a surgeon drills a small opening in the top of the patient's skull and inserts a very small **electrode**. This tiny wire is led

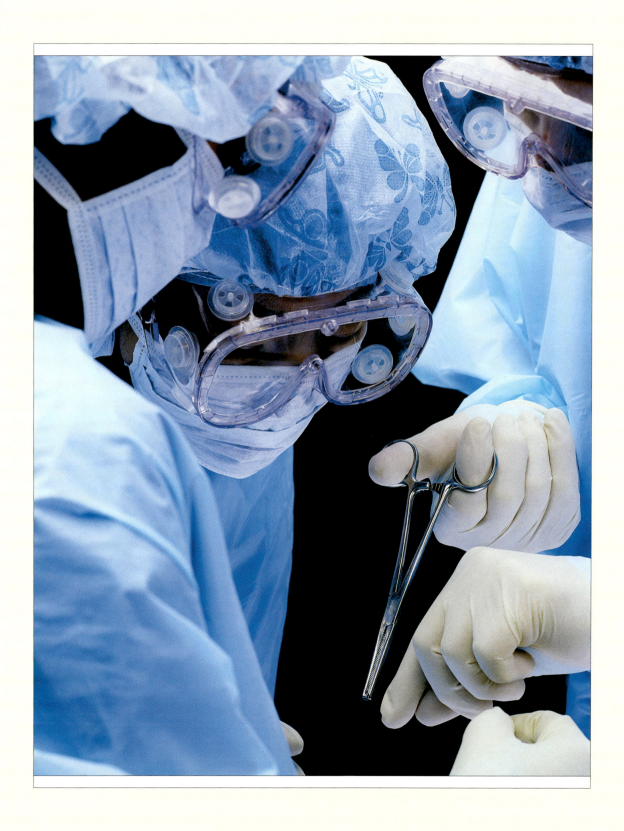

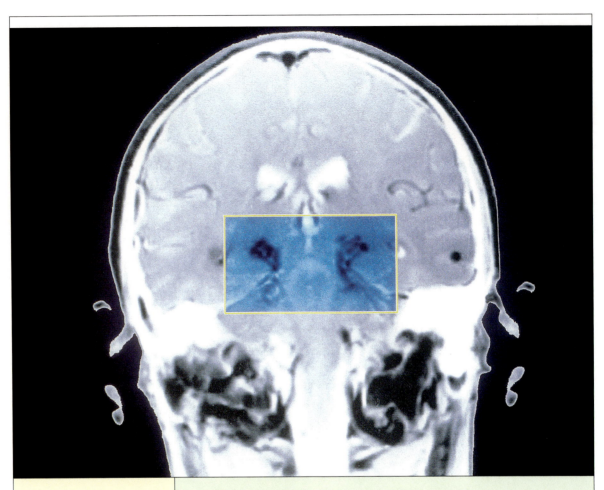

A brain scan pinpoints specific portions of the brain and shows the activities of the neurons.

electrode: a wire through which an electrical current travels

to the area of the brain that causes unwanted movements and destroys its cells. The surgeon must be very careful not to destroy healthy cells, however. This could cause paralysis or partial blindness. If this delicate surgery is successful, the patient usually experiences fewer unwanted movements and less shaking.

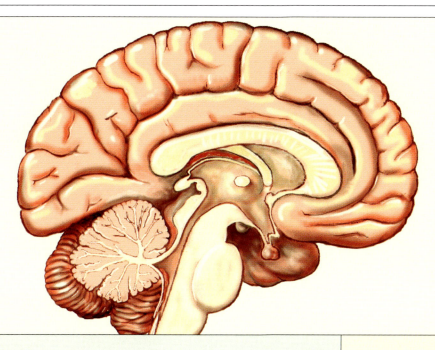

The brain is composed of many distinct sections. Brain surgery often involves removing a small part that is causing problems.

Another brain surgery is called a thalamotomy. Though 90 percent successful, the surgery is a risky one that can result in paralysis, **coma**, or death. In this procedure, the surgeon inserts an electrode into the *thalamus*, a portion of the midbrain that acts as a message center for nerves. A small area of the thalamus is destroyed, eliminating severe **tremors** that normally occur on the left side of the body.

Deep brain stimulation is another option. First, the surgeon permanently places elec-

coma: long-term unconsciousness caused by disease or injury

tremors: involuntary shaking of the body

trodes in the brain. Wires connected to the electrodes are anchored to the inside of the skull. Then the surgeon routes the wires through the base of the skull, past the shoulders, and into the chest area near the collarbone. There, the electrodes are attached to a device similar to a **pacemaker**. Researchers have found that electrical pulses sent to the

pacemaker: an electrical device implanted beneath the skin to regulate a person's heartbeat

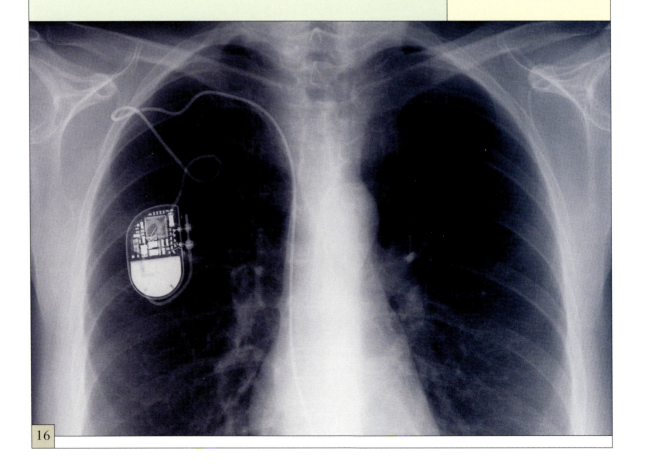

An X-ray image showing a pacemaker in a person's chest. Deep brain stimulation involves the use of a similar device.

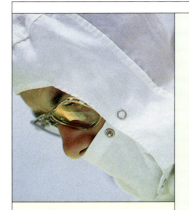

A pallidotomy or thalamotomy is usually considered only as a last option in treating Parkinson's.

neural: relating to the nervous system

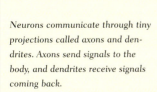

Neurons communicate through tiny projections called axons and dendrites. Axons send signals to the body, and dendrites receive signals coming back.

brain by this device can block the faulty brain signals that cause tremors, a process that scientists call a "jamming of the **neural** network."

According to a study conducted between 1992 and 1997, more than 80 percent of Parkinson's patients had total or significant control of their tremors with deep brain stimulation. Since this procedure does not destroy cells, some patients prefer it to a pallidotomy or a thalamotomy. Most doctors agree that brain surgery is a reasonable option only for patients who are no longer responding to their medication.

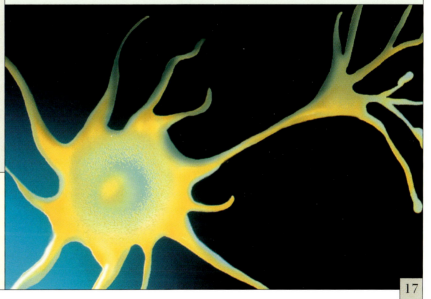

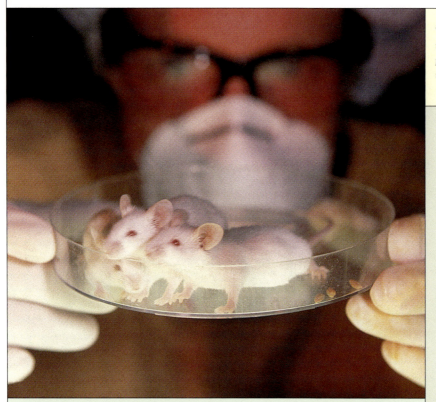

Through their studies with mice, researchers have discovered the possibility of replacing damaged neurons with another type of cell.

stem cells: unspecialized cells that can serve various functions in the body

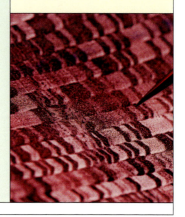

Scientists hope to learn how DNA affects a person's chances of developing Parkinson's.

Scientists are working on ways to make other kinds of human cells produce dopamine. This process is called genetic engineering. Researchers are also testing the effects of injecting neural **stem cells** into the brain. Experiments on mice have shown that this type of cell—when injected into the brain—changes into any type of cell that the damaged brain needs.

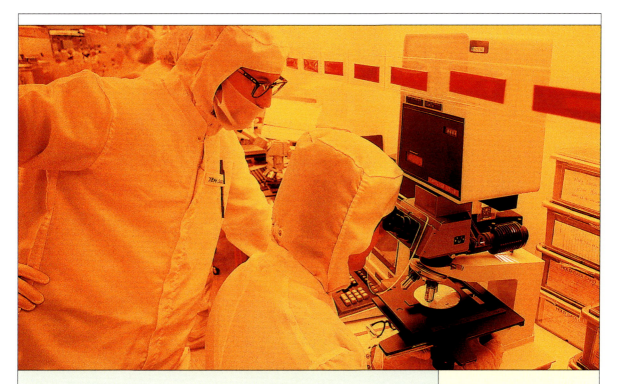

Parkinson's disease was first described nearly 200 years ago, but doctors are still trying to find a cure for it.

Even more importantly, though, researchers are trying to learn why people are struck with Parkinson's disease in the first place. Ultimately, their goal is to find a way to prevent the disease and a way to cure it. In the meantime, new and better ways are being found to help Parkinson's patients go on with their lives.

LIFE GOES ON

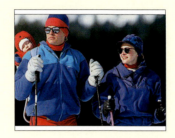

Living with Parkinson's involves changes and challenges. Changes in the body—including muscle stiffness, slower movements, and a stooped posture—can make people with the disease appear older than they are. Facial expressions may become sluggish, causing people to appear sad or uninterested. As physical activities

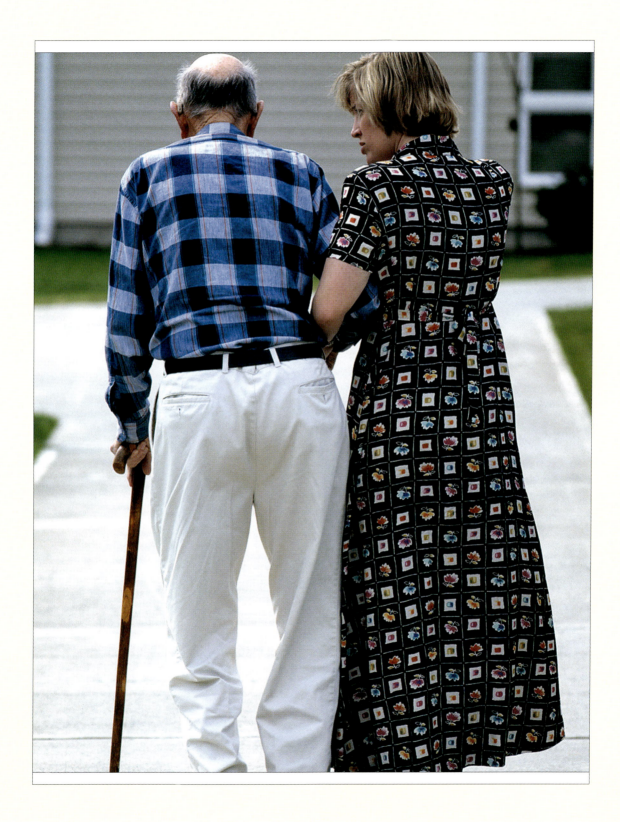

begin to take more effort and energy, people with Parkinson's may find it easier to become inactive. In extreme cases, patients are bed-bound, requiring total care. All of these changes can threaten people's self-esteem and confidence.

Research has shown that depression occurs in about 50 percent of Parkinson's patients. Changes in the chemical makeup of the brain can add to this depression. About 30 percent of

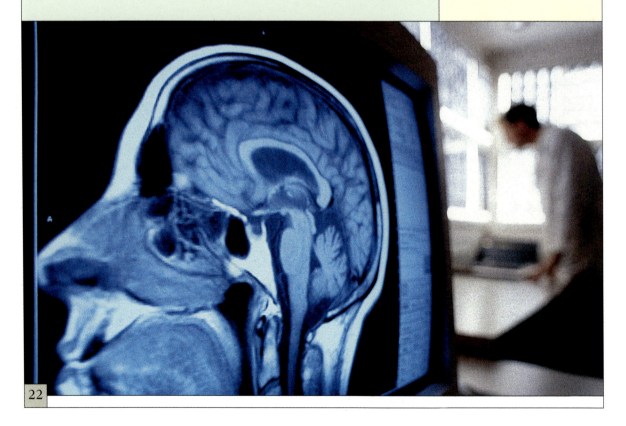

With today's advanced medical facilities, scientists are constantly learning more about the brain's complex functions.

People in advanced stages of Parkinson's disease often need to make adjustments in the type of food they eat.

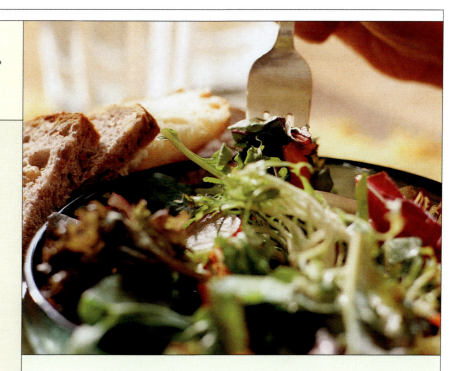

people with Parkinson's also develop some kind of dementia, including the slow loss of memory and intelligence.

Since Parkinson's disease slows down swallowing and the course that food takes through the intestines, people with the illness need to change their eating habits. Frequent, smaller meals are helpful. Levodopa and carbidopa—a common combination of drugs used to treat Parkinson's—work best when taken on an

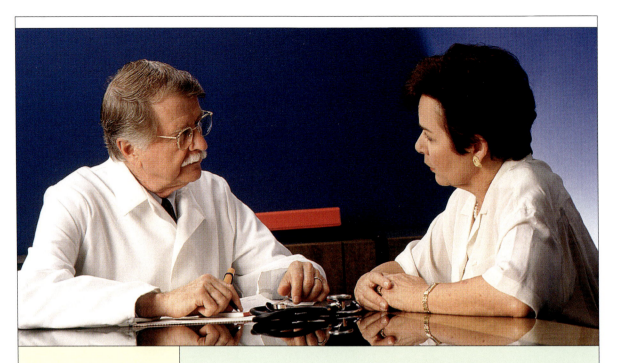

It is important for people with Parkinson's to frequently discuss their symptoms and prescriptions with their doctor.

nausea: a stomach sickness accompanied by an urge to vomit

dehydration: the loss of water or moisture

empty stomach. This allows the drugs to get a head start toward the brain before the body begins digesting food, lessening the treatment's effect. Sometimes taking these drugs without food can cause **nausea**, making it necessary for a person to eat a light snack or take anti-nausea drugs. Drugs taken for Parkinson's can also dry out the body, so it is important to drink plenty of water to avoid **dehydration**.

Lifelong changes and daily challenges can also affect family relationships in unexpected

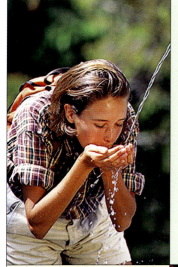

Medication for Parkinson's can cause dehydration, making it necessary to drink lots of water.

ways. Family members may find their activities and social lives altered due to the added responsibility of caring for their loved one. Spouses, children, and caregivers must make changes in the way they live their own lives as they help life go on for the person with

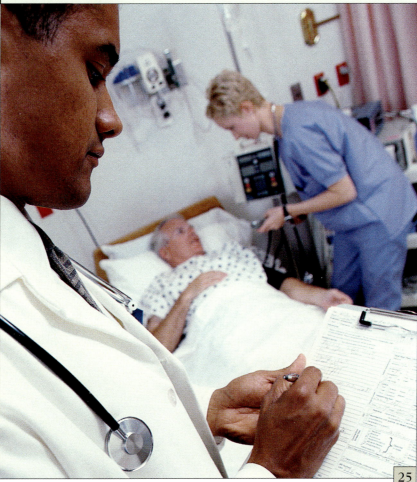

In advanced stages, Parkinson's causes so many problems that patients become bed-bound.

Parkinson's. Employers may need to make adjustments in what they can expect from employees living with the disease. And friends may need to increase their patience and understanding when communication and activities slow down for the person with Parkinson's.

Parkinson's disease does not disrupt only physical movements. It also affects the intellectual, emotional, and social aspects of a person's life. It is a complex disease with many symptoms that are all caused by malfunctioning nerves. Still, with the help of the medical community, support groups, family, and friends, people with Parkinson's can continue to see themselves as valuable human beings and live productive lives. When fears, needs, and concerns are shared, everyone affected by Parkinson's can have the courage to enjoy life, despite the changing circumstances.

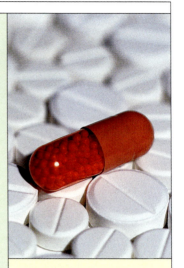

As the disease progresses, Parkinson's patients may need to make many medication adjustments.

Researchers hope to eventually find a cure for Parkinson's by learning more about the brain's nervous system.

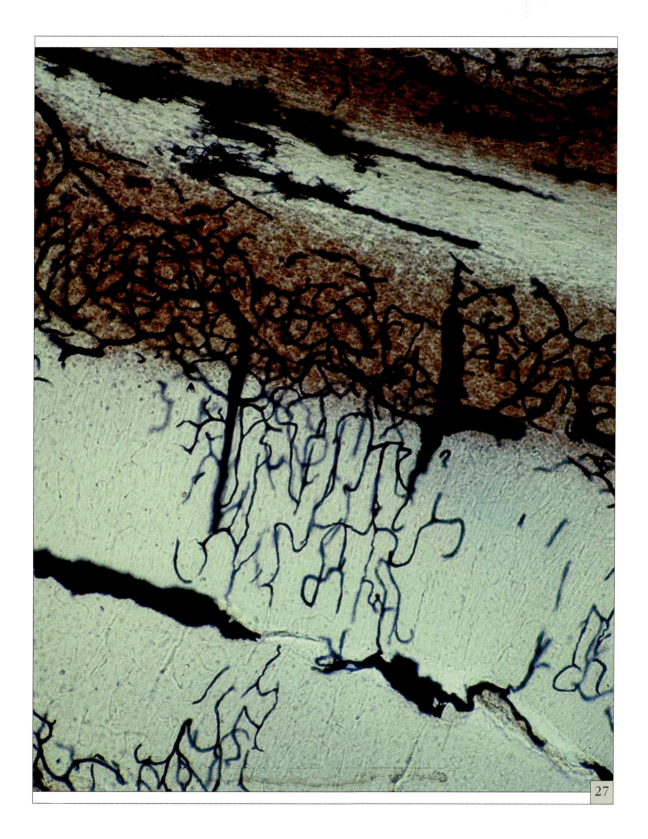

OVERCOMING ILLNESS

Michael J. Fox
ACTOR

MANY PEOPLE RECOGNIZE HIM AS THE TIME-TRAVELING Marty McFly in the *Back to the Future* movies or as Alex P. Keaton in the 1980s hit television series *Family Ties*. But since 1991, Michael J. Fox has had to face a bigger real-life obstacle than anything that he faced in movies or television. That year, while filming a movie, Michael noticed a twitch in his left pinkie finger. Within six months, the tremor spread to his left hand, and his shoulder became stiff. The diagnosis was conclusive: Parkinson's disease.

At first, Michael could not believe that a disease associated with older people could afflict him at the age of 30. Still optimistic, he got second, third, and fourth opinions. All of the doctors agreed with the original diagnosis. For the next few years, the disease progressed until Michael's entire left side was af-

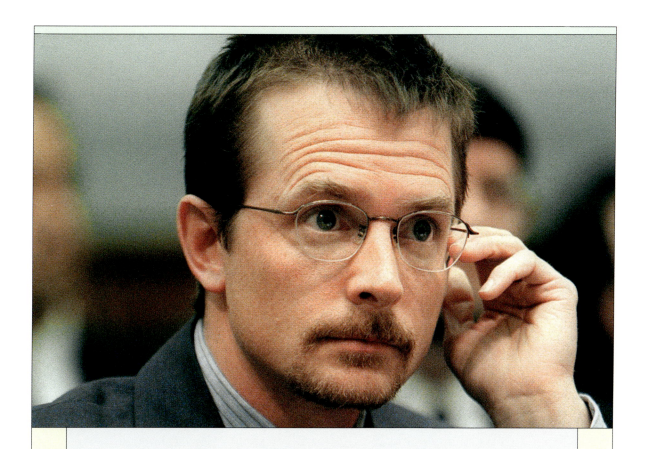

fected by stiffness and uncontrollable shaking. Fine-tuning his medication helped him to continue his career and live a somewhat normal life.

In 1996, Michael took a starring role in the TV series *Spin City*. Two years later, after taping the show's 1998 season finale, Michael went to Holy Family Hospital in Methuen, Massachusetts, to undergo a thalamotomy. The operation was intended to relieve serious tremors by destroying brain cells that were misfiring. The surgery got rid of Michael's worst tremors, but the illness continued to progress.

Michael kept his disease a secret for seven years, confiding only in his family and the *Spin City* cast. But in November 1998, he revealed his illness to the world. Relieved to at last unload his heavy secret, Michael said, "The fact is, I'm seven years down the line with this thing, putting one foot in front of the other, and I haven't mentioned it [to the public]. It might be easier if I did." He said he decided to go public because "I think I can help people by talking."

Realistic about his future, Michael said, "The end is not pretty. I'd like to stop it from its logical conclusion, but I'm grateful. It's made me stronger. A million times wiser. And more compassionate." In his optimistically humorous way, he added, "The biggest thing is that I can be in this situation and still love life as much as I do. Life is great. Sometimes, though, you just have to put up with a little more…."

ORGANIZATIONS

American Parkinson Disease Association, Inc.
1250 Nylan Boulevard, Suite 4B
Staten Island, NY 10305   www.apdaparkinson.com

Movement Disorders Center
Glenbrook and Evanston Hospitals
2100 Pfingsten Road
Glenview, IL 60025

National Parkinson Foundation, Inc.
1501 9th Avenue NW
Bob Hope Road
Miami, FL 33136   www.parkinson.org

The Parkinson Foundation of Canada
National Office
710-390 Bay Street
Toronto, ON   M5H 2Y2

Parkinson's Disease Foundation
William Black Medical Building
Columbia-Presbyterian Medical Center
710 West 168th Street
New York, NY 10032

The Parkinson's Educational Program
3900 Birch Street #105
Newport Beach, CA 92660

The Parkinson's Institute
1170 Morse Avenue
Sunnyvale, CA 94089

United Parkinson Foundation
360 West Superior Street
Chicago, IL 60610

INDEX

A
Ali, Muhammad 10

B
basal ganglia 7–8
brain surgery 12, 14–17, 29–30
  deep brain stimulation 15–17
  pallidotomy 12, 14, 17
  risks 14, 15
  thalamotomy 15, 17, 29–30

D
dementia 23
depression 22
diet 23–24
dopamine 8–9, 11

E
electrodes 12, 14, 15–17

F
Fox, Michael J. 28–30

G
genetic engineering 18

H
Holy Family Hospital 29

M
medication 23–24
  side effects 24

N
nerves 6, 7, 15
neurons 7–8, 17, 26
nigral cells 9–11

P
Parkinson's disease
  causes 4, 9, 10–11
  studies 17–19
  symptoms 4, 9, 20, 22–23, 26, 28–29
  treatments 12, 15–19, 23–24, 29–30

R
Reno, Janet 11

S
stem cells 18
substantia nigra 9

T
thalamus 15

CONTENTS

CHAPTER I 11
    SOME REMARKS ON WITCHCRAFT IN IRELAND

CHAPTER II 23
    A.D. 1324
        DAME ALICE KYTELER, THE SORCERESS OF KILKENNY

CHAPTER III 35
    A.D. 1223-1583
        THE KYTELER CASE AND ITS SURROUNDINGS OF SORCERY AND HERESY—MICHAEL SCOT—THE FOURTH EARL OF DESMOND—JAMES I AND THE IRISH PROPHETESS—A SORCERY ACCUSATION OF 1447—WITCHCRAFT TRIALS IN THE SIXTEENTH CENTURY—STATUTES DEALING WITH THE SUBJECT—EYE-BITERS—THE ENCHANTED EARL OF DESMOND

CHAPTER IV 51
    A.D. 1606-1656
        A CLERICAL WIZARD—WITCHCRAFT CURED BY A RELIC—RAISING THE DEVIL IN IRELAND—HOW HE WAS CHEATED BY A DOCTOR OF DIVINITY—STEWART AND THE FAIRIES—REV. ROBERT BLAIR AND THE MAN POSSESSED WITH A DEVIL—STRANGE OCCURRENCES NEAR LIMERICK—APPARITIONS OF MURDERED

PEOPLE AT PORTADOWN—CHARMED LIVES-VISIONS AND PORTENTS—PETITION OF A BEWITCHED ANTRIM MAN IN ENGLAND—ARCHBISHOP USHER'S PROPHECIES—MR. BROWNE AND THE LOCKED CHEST

CHAPTER V..66
   A.D. 1661
     FLORENCE NEWTON, THE WITCH OF YOUGHAL

CHAPTER VI...79
   A.D. 1662-1686
     THE DEVIL AT DAMERVILLE—AND AT BALLINAGARDE—TAVERNER AND HADDOCK'S GHOST—HUNTER AND THE GHOSTLY OLD WOMAN—A WITCH RESCUED BY THE DEVIL—DR. WILLIAMS AND THE HAUNTED HOUSE IN DUBLIN—APPARITIONS SEEN IN THE AIR IN CO. TIPPERARY—A CLERGYMAN AND HIS WIFE BEWITCHED TO DEATH—BEWITCHING OF MR. MOOR—THE FAIRY-POSSESSED BUTLER—A GHOST INSTIGATES A PROSECUTION—SUPPOSED WITCHCRAFT IN CO. CORK—THE DEVIL AMONG THE QUAKERS.

CHAPTER VII 101
   A.D. 1688
     AN IRISH-AMERICAN WITCH

CHAPTER VIII.. 110
   A.D. 1689-1720
     PORTENT ON ENTRY OF JAMES II—WITCHCRAFT IN CO. ANTRIM—TRADITIONAL VERSION OF SAME—EVENTS PRECEDING THE ISLAND-MAGEE WITCH-TRIAL,—THE TRIAL ITSELF—DR. FRANCIS HUTCHINSON.